RHEUMATOID ARTHRITIS COOKBOOK

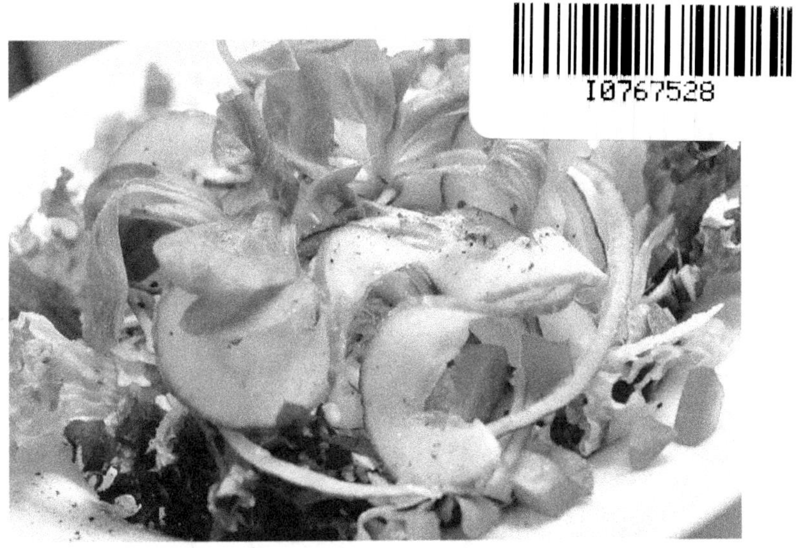

DR. VICKIE STOCK

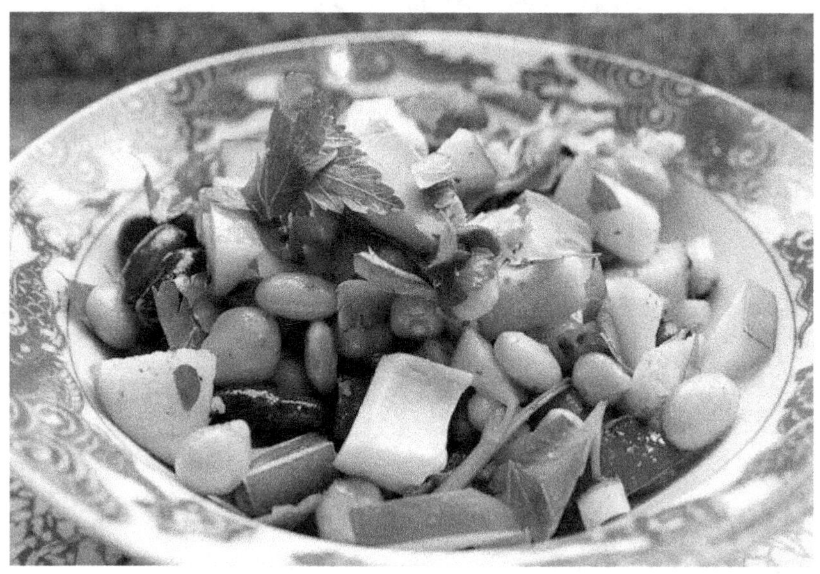

TABLE OF CONTENT

CHAPTER ONE: Understanding Rheumatoid arthritis and Nutrition

Introduction to Rheumatoid Arthritis

Rheumatoid Arthritis (RA) stands as a formidable adversary within the realm of autoimmune diseases, affecting millions of individuals worldwide.

Unlike osteoarthritis, which primarily targets the joints due to wear and tear, rheumatoid arthritis is an autoimmune condition where the body's immune system mistakenly attacks its own tissues, particularly the synovium—the lining of the membranes that surround the joints. This assault triggers a cascade of inflammatory responses, leading to joint pain, swelling, stiffness, and, if left unmanaged, irreversible damage.

The onset of rheumatoid arthritis often occurs in mid-life, typically between the ages of 30 and 60, but it can strike at any age. Women are more frequently affected than men, adding another layer of complexity to this multifaceted condition. While the exact cause remains elusive, a combination of genetic and environmental factors is believed to contribute to its development.

The hallmark of rheumatoid arthritis is its symmetrical pattern of joint involvement, meaning that if one knee or hand is affected, the corresponding one on the other side of the body is likely to be affected as well. Morning stiffness lasting for more than an hour, fatigue, and a general feeling of malaise are common companions to those grappling with RA, making routine activities a daily challenge.

Beyond its impact on joints, rheumatoid arthritis can have systemic effects, affecting organs such as the heart, lungs, and eyes. Early diagnosis and intervention are pivotal in managing the disease effectively, preserving joint function, and mitigating its broader impact on overall health.

As we embark on this culinary journey designed for individuals navigating the complexities of rheumatoid arthritis, the goal is not just to provide nourishing recipes but to empower, inform, and inspire.

Through understanding the intricacies of this autoimmune condition, we can begin to harness the healing potential of a well-balanced, anti-inflammatory diet—one that supports not only the body but also the spirit in the face of rheumatoid arthritis's challenges.

The Role of Nutrition in Managing Rheumatoid Arthritis

Nutrition emerges as a powerful ally in the intricate battle against Rheumatoid Arthritis (RA), offering a unique avenue for managing symptoms and fostering overall well-being. While it cannot provide a cure, a carefully tailored diet can significantly impact the inflammatory processes within the body, alleviating joint pain and stiffness associated with RA.

One cornerstone of an effective nutritional strategy for rheumatoid arthritis revolves around embracing an anti-inflammatory diet. This dietary approach prioritizes foods that possess anti-inflammatory properties, aiming to quell the systemic inflammation at the core of RA.

Omega-3 fatty acids found in fatty fish like salmon, flaxseeds, and walnuts serve as potent anti-inflammatory agents, helping to mitigate the intensity of the immune response.

The incorporation of antioxidants is equally pivotal in managing RA. These compounds, prevalent in fruits and vegetables, combat oxidative stress, a process implicated in the progression of rheumatoid arthritis. Berries, spinach, and kale, with their rich antioxidant profiles, become invaluable additions to a rheumatoid arthritis-friendly menu.

Equally important is understanding the potential impact of certain foods on gut health, considering the intricate connection between the gut and the immune system. Probiotics, found in fermented foods like yogurt and kefir, contribute to a balanced gut microbiome, potentially influencing the course of autoimmune conditions like RA.

Balancing the intake of nutrients, such as maintaining an appropriate level of vitamin D for bone health, is crucial. Collaborating with healthcare professionals to address potential deficiencies ensures a comprehensive and personalized nutritional approach.

The role of nutrition extends beyond mere sustenance—it becomes a proactive measure, a culinary compass guiding individuals toward a path of symptom management and improved quality of life. As we delve into the chapters of this cookbook, we embark on a journey that transcends the kitchen, aiming to empower individuals to harness the transformative potential of their daily food choices in the ongoing quest to conquer rheumatoid arthritis.

Rheumatoid Arthritis (RA) not only affects the joints but also presents a unique set of challenges when it comes to dietary choices. Understanding and navigating these challenges is crucial for individuals seeking to manage their symptoms and optimize their overall health.

One prevalent challenge is the potential for weight fluctuations. RA can impact appetite and metabolism, leading to weight loss or gain. Chronic pain and inflammation may reduce the desire to eat, while certain medications can contribute to weight gain. Striking a balance and maintaining a healthy weight is essential, as excess weight can exacerbate joint stress, while insufficient nutrition may compromise the body's ability to combat inflammation.

Another obstacle is the need to address food sensitivities. Some individuals with rheumatoid arthritis may find certain foods trigger or worsen their symptoms. Common culprits include nightshade vegetables (tomatoes, peppers, eggplants), gluten, and dairy products. Identifying and managing these sensitivities can be challenging but is crucial for personalizing a diet that supports individual health goals.

Dietary challenges also extend to the intersection between RA and bone health. Individuals with RA are at an increased risk of osteoporosis, partly due to the inflammatory nature of the condition and the use of certain medications.

Ensuring an adequate intake of calcium and vitamin D becomes essential for maintaining bone density and minimizing the risk of fractures.

Balancing the nutritional needs for inflammation management is a continuous puzzle for those with rheumatoid arthritis. While anti-inflammatory foods are beneficial, the challenge lies in avoiding pro-inflammatory choices. Processed foods, excessive intake of red meat, and high levels of refined sugars can contribute to inflammation, counteracting the positive effects of an otherwise health-conscious diet.

Navigating these dietary challenges requires a nuanced and personalized approach. Consulting with healthcare professionals, including dietitians and rheumatologists, can provide valuable insights and guidance in crafting a diet that not only addresses the specific needs of rheumatoid arthritis but also promotes overall well-being. By acknowledging and overcoming these challenges, individuals with RA can take proactive steps towards achieving a balanced and supportive relationship between their diet and their health.

Nutritional Goals for Managing Rheumatoid Arthritis

As individuals embark on the journey of managing Rheumatoid Arthritis (RA), setting precise nutritional goals becomes a pivotal aspect of comprehensive care.

While nutrition alone cannot cure RA, it plays a profound role in mitigating symptoms, promoting overall health, and supporting the body's ability to cope with the challenges posed by this autoimmune condition.

One primary nutritional goal for managing RA revolves around reducing inflammation. The anti-inflammatory properties of certain foods can help alleviate joint pain and stiffness. Incorporating omega-3 fatty acids found in fatty fish, flaxseeds, and chia seeds into the diet serves as a potent strategy. These essential fatty acids contribute to the production of anti-inflammatory compounds, offering a natural defense against the persistent inflammation characteristic of RA.

Maintaining a healthy weight stands as another crucial objective. Excess weight places additional stress on joints, exacerbating RA symptoms. Balanced nutrition, combined with regular exercise, not only aids in weight management but also contributes to improved joint function and overall well-being.

Supporting bone health is an essential nutritional goal, as individuals with RA are at an increased risk of osteoporosis. Adequate calcium and vitamin D intake through dairy products, leafy greens, and fortified foods becomes imperative in preserving bone density and preventing fractures.

Balancing macronutrients is vital for energy and immune support. A diet rich in lean proteins, whole grains, and a variety of fruits and vegetables ensures a diverse array of essential nutrients. Protein plays a crucial role in muscle maintenance, supporting individuals in maintaining strength and mobility despite the challenges posed by RA.

Hydration should not be overlooked, as proper fluid intake contributes to joint lubrication and overall health. Water, herbal teas, and nutrient-rich fluids should be prioritized over sugary or caffeinated beverages.

Individualizing these nutritional goals in consultation with healthcare professionals ensures a tailored approach that considers the specific needs and sensitivities of each person managing RA. By incorporating these nutritional goals into their daily lives, individuals can take proactive steps toward enhancing their quality of life and effectively managing the impact of Rheumatoid Arthritis.

Building a Supportive Dietary Foundation for Rheumatoid Arthritis

Creating a dietary foundation that supports individuals grappling with Rheumatoid Arthritis (RA) involves a strategic blend of nutrient-rich foods, mindful choices, and a holistic approach to overall well-being. This foundation serves as a cornerstone for managing symptoms, promoting joint health, and enhancing the quality of life for those navigating the challenges of RA.

A key aspect of this supportive dietary foundation is the emphasis on whole, unprocessed foods. Fruits, vegetables, whole grains, and lean proteins form the building blocks, providing a diverse array of vitamins, minerals, antioxidants, and essential nutrients. These foods not only nourish the body but also contribute to a balanced and anti-inflammatory environment, crucial for mitigating the effects of RA.

Incorporating a rainbow of colors on the plate becomes a guiding principle. Different hues signify distinct phytonutrients and antioxidants, each playing a unique role in promoting health.

Deeply colored berries, leafy greens, and vibrant vegetables contribute to the overall anti-inflammatory and immune-boosting potential of the diet.

Omega-3 fatty acids, renowned for their anti-inflammatory properties, are integral to the dietary foundation for RA. Fatty fish like salmon, walnuts, and flaxseeds provide abundant sources of these essential fats, offering a natural defense against the chronic inflammation characteristic of the condition.

Mindful eating practices are interwoven into the fabric of this dietary foundation. Savoring each bite, paying attention to hunger and fullness cues, and cultivating an awareness of how different foods impact the body fosters a positive relationship with food. Additionally, recognizing potential food sensitivities and making informed choices regarding dietary exclusions can contribute to a more personalized and effective approach to managing RA symptoms.

Hydration remains a fundamental component, with water being the primary beverage of choice. Staying well-hydrated is essential for joint lubrication, toxin elimination, and overall bodily functions.

CHAPTER TWO: Anti-inflammatory foods for Rheumatoid arthritis

Introduction to Anti-Inflammatory Diet

The concept of an anti-inflammatory diet has gained significant traction as a proactive and empowering approach to managing various health conditions, including inflammatory disorders like Rheumatoid Arthritis (RA). At its core, the anti-inflammatory diet is not just a temporary eating plan but a lifestyle that focuses on consuming foods with the potential to mitigate chronic inflammation—the underlying culprit in many health challenges.

Central to this dietary approach is the incorporation of foods rich in anti-inflammatory properties. Omega-3 fatty acids found in fatty fish like salmon, flaxseeds, and walnuts are key players in the fight against inflammation. These essential fats serve as precursors to anti-inflammatory compounds, aiding in the modulation of the body's inflammatory response.

Herbs and spices also take center stage in the anti-inflammatory diet. Turmeric, with its active component curcumin, boasts potent anti-inflammatory and antioxidant properties. Ginger, cinnamon, and garlic are additional culinary allies known for their anti-inflammatory benefits, enhancing both flavor and health in meals.

Fruits and vegetables, particularly those rich in antioxidants, play a pivotal role. Berries, leafy greens, and colorful vegetables contribute a spectrum of vitamins, minerals, and phytonutrients that combat oxidative stress and inflammation. These plant-based powerhouses form the foundation of an anti-inflammatory plate.

Whole grains and legumes round out the diet, providing fiber and essential nutrients. Fiber not only supports gut health but also helps regulate blood sugar levels, reducing the risk of inflammatory responses associated with elevated blood sugar.

The anti-inflammatory diet is more than just a list of foods to include; it's about creating a harmonious balance and synergy among these nutrient-dense choices. While it may not replace medical treatments, adopting an anti-inflammatory lifestyle, in collaboration with healthcare professionals, can be a potent tool in managing conditions like RA.

Omega-3 Fatty Acids and Their Role in Joint Health

Omega-3 fatty acids stand as unsung heroes in the realm of nutrition, particularly when it comes to joint health. Among the three main types of omega-3s—eicosapentaenoic acid (EPA), docosahexaenoic acid (DHA), and alpha-linolenic acid (ALA)—EPA and DHA, primarily found in fatty fish and certain algae, have garnered attention for their profound impact on maintaining healthy joints.

These essential fatty acids play a pivotal role in reducing inflammation, a key factor in joint pain and stiffness associated with conditions like Rheumatoid Arthritis (RA). In the inflammatory cascade, omega-3s act as precursors to specialized molecules called eicosanoids, which exert anti-inflammatory effects.

By promoting the synthesis of these anti-inflammatory compounds, omega-3 fatty acids help temper the overactive immune response often seen in inflammatory joint conditions.

Furthermore, the lubrication of joints is crucial for smooth movement and flexibility. Omega-3s contribute to joint lubrication by supporting the production of synovial fluid, a viscous liquid that nourishes and cushions the joints.

This lubrication mechanism is particularly vital in mitigating the friction and wear-and-tear on joints, fostering their overall health and functionality.

Scientific studies have demonstrated the efficacy of omega-3 supplementation in reducing the severity of joint pain and morning stiffness in individuals with rheumatoid arthritis.

Incorporating omega-3-rich foods, such as salmon, mackerel, sardines, and flaxseeds, into the diet becomes a strategic and delicious way to harness the joint-protective benefits of these fatty acids.

While omega-3 fatty acids are not a cure for joint conditions, they offer a natural and complementary approach to managing symptoms and supporting overall joint health.

Incorporating Turmeric and Other Anti-Inflammatory Spices

Within the vibrant tapestry of culinary delights, spices like turmeric emerge not only as flavor enhancers but also as potent allies in the quest for health and wellness. Turmeric, renowned for its active compound curcumin, stands out prominently among anti-inflammatory spices, offering a spectrum of benefits, especially in the context of managing conditions like Rheumatoid Arthritis (RA).

Curcumin, the golden-hued magic within turmeric, boasts powerful anti-inflammatory and antioxidant properties. It has been the focus of numerous studies exploring its potential to alleviate joint pain and stiffness associated with inflammatory conditions.

Including turmeric in the diet is not only a flavorful choice but a strategic one for those seeking to harness the anti-inflammatory benefits nature has to offer.

Pairing turmeric with black pepper enhances its bioavailability, ensuring that the body can absorb and utilize curcumin more effectively. This dynamic duo becomes a culinary powerhouse, easily incorporated into various dishes, from curries to soups, imparting both flavor and potential health benefits.

Beyond turmeric, an array of anti-inflammatory spices adds depth and complexity to dishes while contributing to overall well-being. Ginger, with its zesty and warming notes, shares anti-inflammatory and analgesic properties, potentially easing joint discomfort.

Cinnamon, not just a delightful sweetener, has been linked to reducing inflammation and oxidative stress. Cayenne pepper, with its fiery kick, contains capsaicin, renowned for its anti-inflammatory effects.

Incorporating these spices into daily meals becomes a culinary adventure, where each sprinkle and dash contributes not only to the palate but also to the body's resilience. From savory stews to comforting teas, the canvas for incorporating anti-inflammatory spices is vast and versatile.

Benefits of Berries and Other Antioxidant-Rich Foods

Berries and other antioxidant-rich foods emerge as nutritional powerhouses, offering an array of benefits that extend far beyond their delightful flavors. For individuals navigating conditions like Rheumatoid Arthritis (RA), these vibrant foods play a pivotal role in supporting overall health and combating inflammation.

Berries, such as blueberries, strawberries, raspberries, and blackberries, are brimming with antioxidants, including flavonoids and polyphenols. These compounds act as scavengers for free radicals—unstable molecules that contribute to oxidative stress and inflammation in the body. By neutralizing these free radicals, berries play a crucial role in mitigating the inflammatory processes associated with RA.

Beyond berries, a spectrum of antioxidant-rich foods contributes to the body's defense against inflammation. Dark leafy greens, like kale and spinach, are rich in vitamins A, C, and K, as well as various antioxidants.

Nuts and seeds, particularly walnuts and flaxseeds, provide a potent dose of omega-3 fatty acids alongside their antioxidant content, offering a dual-action approach to inflammation management.

Colorful vegetables, such as bell peppers, tomatoes, and sweet potatoes, are not only visually appealing but also rich sources of antioxidants like vitamin C and beta-carotene. These nutrients contribute to the body's ability to repair and regenerate tissues, supporting joint health and overall well-being.

The benefits of incorporating antioxidant-rich foods extend beyond their anti-inflammatory properties. They contribute to the maintenance of a robust immune system, enhance cardiovascular health, and support cellular integrity. Including a variety of these foods in the daily diet becomes a delicious and proactive strategy for individuals with RA, offering a symphony of flavors and nutrients that nourish both the body and the spirit.

Meal Plans and Recipes to Reduce Inflammation

Crafting meal plans and recipes to reduce inflammation becomes a dynamic and flavorful strategy for individuals seeking relief from conditions like Rheumatoid Arthritis (RA).

A thoughtful and intentional approach to food can harness the anti-inflammatory potential of various ingredients, creating a symphony of flavors that not only tantalize the taste buds but also nourish the body.

The foundation of an anti-inflammatory meal plan revolves around incorporating whole, nutrient-dense foods. Fruits and vegetables, particularly those rich in antioxidants, such as berries, leafy greens, and colorful vegetables, take center stage.

These foods contribute essential vitamins, minerals, and phytonutrients that combat oxidative stress and dampen the flames of inflammation.

Fatty fish, like salmon, mackerel, and sardines, bring a generous dose of omega-3 fatty acids to the table. These essential fats, with their anti-inflammatory properties, become a cornerstone for joint health and overall well-being. Nuts, seeds, and olive oil further contribute to the healthy fat profile of the meal plan.

Whole grains, such as quinoa, brown rice, and oats, provide fiber and a variety of nutrients, offering sustained energy while supporting gut health. Legumes, rich in protein and fiber, become versatile additions, promoting satiety and contributing to a balanced diet.

Spices like turmeric, ginger, and cinnamon add depth and anti-inflammatory benefits to dishes. These culinary delights not only elevate the flavor profile but also infuse meals with a natural defense against inflammation.

Sample recipes might include a quinoa salad with mixed berries and walnuts, a grilled salmon dish with a turmeric and ginger marinade, or a vibrant vegetable stir-fry featuring an array of colorful produce.

These recipes showcase the diversity and creativity inherent in an anti-inflammatory meal plan, proving that eating to reduce inflammation can be both delicious and satisfying.

In the journey towards managing RA through nutrition, meal plans and recipes become more than nourishment; they become tools for empowerment and well-being. As individuals embrace the flavors and healing potential of these culinary creations, they embark on a path that intertwines the joy of eating with the pursuit of a healthier, more vibrant life.

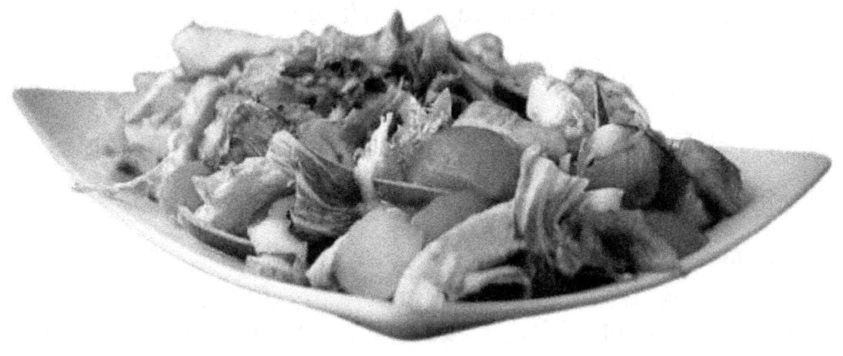

CHAPTER THREE: Bone Health and Rheumatoid Arthritis

Importance of Bone Health in Rheumatoid Arthritis

Importance of Bone Health in Rheumatoid Arthritis

In the intricate landscape of Rheumatoid Arthritis (RA), where the focus often centers on joint inflammation and pain, the significance of bone health should not be overlooked.

RA not only affects the synovium—the lining of joints—but can also exert a profound impact on bone density and integrity, posing additional challenges for those navigating this autoimmune condition.

The chronic inflammation characteristic of RA can lead to the erosion of cartilage and bone tissue. As the disease progresses, this process may escalate, resulting in joint deformities and bone damage. Moreover, the use of certain medications, such as glucocorticoids, commonly prescribed to manage RA symptoms, can further contribute to bone loss.

Osteoporosis, a condition characterized by weakened and porous bones, becomes a heightened concern for individuals with RA. The increased risk of fractures is not only attributed to the direct impact of inflammation on bone but also to the potential side effects of medications and the challenges posed by reduced physical activity due to joint pain.

Maintaining optimal bone health thus becomes a crucial aspect of managing RA comprehensively. Adequate intake of calcium and vitamin D, essential for bone strength and calcium absorption, should be prioritized. Incorporating dairy products, leafy greens, and fortified foods into the diet can help meet these nutritional needs.

Weight-bearing exercises, adapted to individual abilities and joint conditions, play a dual role in supporting bone health and maintaining joint function. Strengthening exercises contribute to bone density, while weight-bearing activities such as walking or low-impact aerobics can be tailored to promote overall fitness without exacerbating joint stress.

For Rheumatoid Arthritis management, addressing bone health is a proactive step towards sustaining the structural integrity of the skeletal system. A multidimensional approach that encompasses nutrition, exercise, and medication management, in collaboration with healthcare professionals, offers a holistic strategy for preserving bone health and enhancing the overall quality of life for individuals navigating the complexities of RA.

Calcium and Vitamin D for Joint and Bone Support

The factors influencing joint and bone health, calcium and vitamin D stand out as dynamic duo essential for maintaining skeletal strength and resilience.

For individuals grappling with conditions like Rheumatoid Arthritis (RA), where the risk of bone density loss is heightened, ensuring an adequate supply of these nutrients becomes a crucial component of comprehensive management. Calcium, often lauded for its role in bone formation and density, is a mineral vital for the structural integrity of the skeletal system.

Bones act as a reservoir for calcium, releasing and absorbing the mineral as needed. In the context of RA, where chronic inflammation can contribute to bone loss, ensuring an adequate intake of calcium becomes pivotal for preserving bone density and preventing fractures.

Vitamin D, the "sunshine vitamin," complements calcium's efforts by facilitating its absorption in the intestines. Beyond this crucial partnership, vitamin D plays a multifaceted role in immune function and inflammatory regulation, making it particularly relevant for individuals with RA. Exposure to sunlight remains a natural source of vitamin D, while dietary sources include fatty fish, fortified dairy products, and vitamin D supplements when necessary.

The synergy between calcium and vitamin D becomes especially pronounced in supporting joint health. RA's inflammatory processes can impact the synovium and surrounding tissues, exacerbating joint pain and stiffness. A well-maintained skeletal system provides a robust framework that better withstands the challenges posed by inflammation, contributing to overall joint function.

Foods That Promote Bone Strength

Nurturing bone strength is a multifaceted endeavor, and the role of nutrition cannot be overstated, especially for those managing conditions like Rheumatoid Arthritis (RA). Incorporating a variety of nutrient-rich foods into the diet can significantly contribute to bone health, providing the essential building blocks necessary for maintaining skeletal strength and resilience.

➢ Dairy Products: Known for their rich calcium content, dairy products such as milk, yogurt, and cheese are fundamental contributors to bone strength. Calcium is a primary mineral in bones, and its adequate intake is vital for maintaining bone density.

➢ Leafy Greens: Dark, leafy greens like kale, collard greens, and spinach are not only abundant in calcium but also provide additional nutrients like vitamin K, which plays a role in bone metabolism and mineralization.

➢ Fatty Fish: Salmon, mackerel, and sardines are not only excellent sources of omega-3 fatty acids but also contribute to bone health. These fatty acids support calcium absorption and may have anti-inflammatory effects beneficial for individuals managing RA.

➢ Fortified Foods: Many foods, including certain plant-based milk alternatives and breakfast cereals, are fortified with calcium and vitamin D. These fortified options offer flexibility for individuals with dietary restrictions or preferences.

➢ Nuts and Seeds: Almonds, chia seeds, and sesame seeds are rich in calcium and provide additional nutrients like magnesium and phosphorus, contributing to overall bone health.

➢ Fortified Tofu: Tofu, a staple in many vegetarian and vegan diets, can be fortified with calcium and is an excellent plant-based option for supporting bone strength.

➢ Bone Broth: Rich in minerals like calcium, magnesium, and phosphorus, bone broth offers a nourishing option that can be incorporated into soups and stews for added flavor and bone-boosting benefits.

Strategies for Maintaining Bone Density

Maintaining optimal bone density is a critical aspect of overall health, particularly for individuals managing conditions such as Rheumatoid Arthritis (RA). As chronic inflammation and certain medications associated with RA can pose challenges to bone health, adopting proactive strategies becomes paramount in preserving skeletal strength and resilience.

- Adequate Calcium Intake: Calcium is the cornerstone of bone health, contributing to bone density and strength.

- Ensuring an adequate intake of calcium through dietary sources such as dairy products, leafy greens, and fortified foods is essential. For those with dietary restrictions or preferences, calcium supplements may be considered under the guidance of healthcare professionals.

- Vitamin D Supplementation: Vitamin D plays a pivotal role in calcium absorption and bone metabolism. Sunlight exposure remains a natural source of vitamin D, but individuals with limited sun exposure or absorption issues may benefit from vitamin D supplements to maintain optimal levels.

- Regular Weight-Bearing Exercise: Weight-bearing exercises, such as walking, jogging, and resistance training, are instrumental in stimulating bone formation and maintaining bone density.

Tailoring exercise regimens to individual capabilities and consulting with healthcare professionals ensures a safe and effective approach.

➢ Balanced Nutrition: Beyond calcium and vitamin D, a well-rounded diet that includes a variety of nutrients, such as magnesium, phosphorus, and vitamin K, supports overall bone health. Dark, leafy greens, nuts, seeds, and fatty fish are valuable additions to a bone-friendly diet.

➢ Limiting Alcohol and Caffeine: Excessive alcohol consumption and high caffeine intake have been associated with bone loss. Moderation in alcohol consumption and mindful consumption of caffeinated beverages contribute to bone health.

➢ Quit Smoking: Smoking has detrimental effects on bone health, leading to decreased bone density and increased fracture risk. Quitting smoking not only benefits overall health but also positively impacts bone strength.

➢ Regular Bone Density Monitoring: For individuals with RA or other risk factors for bone density loss, regular monitoring through bone density scans helps assess the effectiveness of preventive measures and allows for timely intervention if needed.

CHAPTER FOUR: Maintaining a Healthy Weight with Rheumatoid Arthritis

Weight Management and Its Impact on Joint Health

The intricate relationship between weight management and joint health becomes particularly pronounced in conditions such as Rheumatoid Arthritis (RA), where joints already face the challenge of chronic inflammation. Maintaining a healthy weight is a proactive strategy that significantly influences joint function, potentially alleviating pain and enhancing overall well-being.

Excess body weight places additional stress on joints, especially weight-bearing ones like the knees and hips. For individuals with RA, where inflammation already contributes to joint discomfort, the added burden of excess weight can exacerbate symptoms. Engaging in weight management strategies becomes crucial in mitigating this impact.

➢ Reduced Joint Stress: Every pound of excess weight translates to increased stress on weight-bearing joints. By shedding extra pounds, individuals can reduce the load on their joints, diminishing wear-and-tear and potentially slowing down the progression of joint damage.

➢ Inflammation Control: Adipose tissue, commonly known as fat, is not merely a passive store of energy. It actively produces inflammatory substances, contributing to systemic inflammation.

Weight management, through a combination of healthy eating and regular exercise, can help regulate inflammation, providing relief for individuals with RA.

➢ Improved Medication Efficacy: Weight management can positively impact the effectiveness of medications used to manage RA symptoms. Achieving and maintaining a healthy weight may enhance the response to treatment, allowing for better control of inflammation and joint pain.

➢ Enhanced Joint Function: A healthy weight promotes improved joint function. Reduced joint stress and inflammation contribute to enhanced mobility and flexibility, allowing individuals to engage in physical activities that support joint health without exacerbating symptoms.

Adopting a holistic approach to weight management involves a balanced diet, regular physical activity, and lifestyle modifications. Consulting with healthcare professionals, including rheumatologists and nutritionists, ensures personalized strategies tailored to individual needs and conditions.

By recognizing the intimate connection between weight management and joint health, individuals with RA can empower themselves to actively contribute to the well-being of their joints. The journey towards a healthy weight becomes not only a means of achieving physical vitality but also a proactive step towards managing the complexities of RA with resilience and empowerment.

In the pursuit of weight control, the key lies not in deprivation but in fostering a harmonious relationship with food through balanced nutrition. Striking the right balance ensures that the body receives essential nutrients while managing caloric intake, offering a sustainable approach to weight management that is both effective and nourishing.

> ➤ Nutrient-Rich Foods: Prioritize nutrient-dense foods that provide a wealth of vitamins, minerals, and antioxidants without excessive calories. Include colorful fruits and vegetables, lean proteins, whole grains, and healthy fats in your daily meals. These foods not only contribute to overall well-being but also support weight control by promoting satiety and reducing the likelihood of overeating.

> ➤ Protein for Satiety: Including lean protein sources, such as poultry, fish, tofu, and legumes, is crucial for weight control. Protein not only supports muscle health but also promotes a feeling of fullness, reducing the temptation to indulge in unhealthy snacks between meals.

> ➤ Whole Grains and Fiber: Opt for whole grains like brown rice, quinoa, and whole wheat bread, along with fiber-rich foods such as fruits, vegetables, and legumes. Fiber enhances satiety, aids in digestion, and helps control blood sugar levels, contributing to weight management.

> ➤ Mindful Eating: Cultivate mindful eating habits by savoring each bite, paying attention to hunger and fullness cues, and avoiding

distractions during meals. Mindful eating fosters a deeper connection with food, preventing overconsumption and promoting a healthier relationship with eating.

➢ Hydration: Staying well-hydrated is essential for overall health and can support weight control. Often, the body may mistake thirst for hunger, leading to unnecessary calorie consumption. Drinking water throughout the day helps maintain hydration and may contribute to a sense of fullness.

➢ Moderation and Variety: Embrace the philosophy of moderation, allowing yourself occasional treats without guilt. Variety in your diet ensures a broad spectrum of nutrients, making it easier to adhere to a balanced and sustainable eating plan.

Achieving and maintaining weight control is not about restrictive diets but about adopting a lifestyle that prioritizes balanced nutrition. Consulting with registered dietitians or nutritionists can provide personalized guidance, ensuring that nutritional needs are met while supporting the journey towards a healthier weight and overall well-being.

Exercise and Physical Activity for Rheumatoid Arthritis Patients

Engaging in regular exercise and physical activity is a cornerstone of comprehensive care for individuals with Rheumatoid Arthritis (RA). Despite the challenges posed by joint pain and stiffness, adopting a tailored and well-monitored exercise routine offers a myriad of benefits, contributing to improved joint function, increased strength, and enhanced overall well-being.

- ➢ Joint Mobility and Flexibility: RA often leads to decreased joint mobility and stiffness. Incorporating exercises that focus on joint range of motion, such as gentle stretching and yoga, can help alleviate stiffness and maintain flexibility. These activities improve joint function, making daily tasks more manageable.

- ➢ Strengthening Exercises: Strengthening the muscles surrounding affected joints is crucial for individuals with RA. Targeted strength training, using resistance bands or light weights under the guidance of a physiotherapist or exercise specialist, helps stabilize joints and reduces the risk of deformities.

- ➢ Low-Impact Cardiovascular Exercise: Low-impact cardiovascular exercises, such as swimming, walking, or stationary cycling, provide cardiovascular benefits without putting excessive stress on the joints. Regular aerobic exercise contributes to overall fitness, helps manage weight, and promotes a healthy heart.

- ➢ Balance and Stability Training: RA can affect balance and stability, increasing the risk of falls. Incorporating exercises that focus on balance, such as tai chi, can enhance stability and reduce the likelihood of accidents. Balance training is especially important for maintaining independence and preventing injuries.

- ➢ Pacing and Adaptations: Understanding individual limitations and adopting a pacing approach to exercise is essential for individuals with RA.

- ➢ Breaking activities into manageable segments, allowing for rest when needed, and using adaptive tools or techniques ensure a safe and sustainable exercise routine.
- ➢ Mind-Body Practices: Mind-body practices, including meditation and relaxation techniques, can complement physical activities by reducing stress and promoting a positive mindset. Stress management is crucial for individuals with RA, as stress can exacerbate symptoms.

Before starting any exercise program, it is crucial for individuals with RA to consult with their healthcare team, including rheumatologists and physiotherapists. Tailoring exercise plans to individual needs and gradually progressing in intensity helps ensure a safe and effective approach to physical activity, empowering individuals with RA to actively manage their condition and lead a more vibrant and resilient life.

Mindful Eating Strategies

In a world often characterized by fast-paced lifestyles and hectic schedules, cultivating mindful eating habits offers a transformative approach to nourishing the body, fostering a healthier relationship with food, and promoting overall well-being.

Mindful eating involves paying full attention to the sensory experience of eating, acknowledging hunger and fullness cues, and savoring each bite. Here are some mindful eating strategies to incorporate into daily life:

- Eat with Awareness: Begin meals by taking a moment to appreciate the appearance, aroma, and textures of the food on your plate. Engage your senses fully in the experience, creating a mindful environment that enhances the pleasure of eating.

- Slow Down: Eating at a slower pace allows the body to register satiety cues more effectively. Put down utensils between bites, chew food thoroughly, and savor the flavors. This not only aids digestion but also fosters a sense of contentment with smaller portions.

- Listen to Your Body: Tune into your body's hunger and fullness signals. Eat when you're genuinely hungry, and stop when you feel satisfied. Avoid eating out of boredom, stress, or other emotional triggers by checking in with your body's true needs.

- Mindful Portion Control: Be mindful of portion sizes, and avoid the temptation to mindlessly consume large quantities. Using smaller plates, bowls, and utensils can help create a visual illusion of a fuller plate while promoting portion control.

- Limit Distractions: Minimize distractions during meals by turning off electronic devices, stepping away from work, and creating a dedicated eating space. This allows you to focus on the act of eating and fully enjoy your food.

- Embrace Gratitude: Take a moment to express gratitude for your meal. Reflect on the journey of the food from its source to your plate, fostering a sense of appreciation for the nourishment it provides.

> Recognize Emotional Eating: Be aware of emotional triggers that may lead to mindless eating. Instead of turning to food for comfort, explore alternative coping mechanisms such as deep breathing, meditation, or engaging in activities that bring joy.

Weight Management Meal Plans and Recipes

Crafting a weight management meal plan involves a thoughtful and balanced approach that prioritizes nutrient-rich foods while controlling caloric intake. Here are some key principles and delectable recipes designed to support weight management:

Principles of Weight Management Meal Plans:

> Balanced Macronutrients: Include a combination of lean proteins, complex carbohydrates, and healthy fats in each meal. This balance helps maintain energy levels, promotes satiety, and supports overall nutritional needs.
>
> Portion Control: Be mindful of portion sizes to avoid overeating. Using smaller plates and bowls can create an optical illusion of a fuller plate, assisting in portion control.
>
> Fiber-Rich Foods: Incorporate fiber-rich foods like fruits, vegetables, whole grains, and legumes. Fiber promotes feelings of fullness, aids in digestion, and helps regulate blood sugar levels.
>
> Hydration: Stay well-hydrated throughout the day. Drinking water before meals can contribute to a sense of fullness, potentially reducing overall calorie intake.
>
> Meal Frequency: Consider smaller, frequent meals to help regulate metabolism and prevent extreme hunger, which may lead to overeating.

CHAPTER FIVE: Practical Tips for Everyday Cooking and Dining

Grocery Shopping Tips and Ingredient Substitutions

Navigating the aisles of a grocery store with a focus on health and mindful choices can significantly impact your overall well-being. Here are some grocery shopping tips and ingredient substitutions to foster a nutritious and balanced approach to food selection:

Grocery Shopping Tips:

➢ Plan Ahead: Create a shopping list based on your meal plans for the week. This helps you stay focused, avoid impulse purchases, and ensures you have the ingredients needed for balanced meals.

➢ Shop the Perimeter: The perimeter of the grocery store typically houses fresh produce, lean proteins, and dairy. Prioritize these sections for wholesome, unprocessed options.

➢ Read Labels: Be mindful of ingredient lists and nutritional labels. Choose items with minimal additives, lower sodium content, and limited added sugars. Look for whole, recognizable ingredients.

➢ Choose Whole Grains: Opt for whole grains like brown rice, quinoa, and whole wheat bread instead of refined grains. Whole grains offer more nutrients and fiber, contributing to satiety and overall health.

➢ Include a Variety of Colors: A colorful shopping cart often signifies a diverse array of nutrients.

- ➢ Incorporate a rainbow of fruits and vegetables to ensure a broad spectrum of vitamins and minerals.

Ingredient Substitutions:

- ➢ Greek Yogurt for Sour Cream: Substitute Greek yogurt for sour cream in recipes for a lower-fat and higher-protein alternative. It works well in dips, dressings, and baked goods.
- ➢ Cauliflower Rice for Regular Rice: Replace traditional rice with cauliflower rice to lower calorie and carbohydrate content while increasing vegetable intake. It's a versatile option for various dishes.
- ➢ Avocado for Butter: Use mashed avocado in place of butter in baking or as a spread for a heart-healthy alternative rich in monounsaturated fats.
- ➢ Spaghetti Squash for Pasta: Swap pasta with spaghetti squash for a low-carb, vegetable-based alternative. Top with your favorite sauce or incorporate into casseroles for added nutrients.
- ➢ Almond Flour for All-Purpose Flour: Almond flour serves as a gluten-free and higher-protein substitute for all-purpose flour in baking recipes. It imparts a nutty flavor and a moist texture.

By incorporating these grocery shopping tips and ingredient substitutions into your routine, you not only make informed choices at the store but also foster a flexible and health-conscious approach to cooking. These small adjustments contribute to a more mindful and satisfying culinary experience while supporting your overall health goals.

Navigating restaurant menus with Rheumatoid Arthritis (RA) involves thoughtful consideration to ensure an enjoyable dining experience while accommodating the unique challenges posed by joint inflammation and stiffness. Here are some dining-out strategies tailored to the needs of individuals with RA:

➢ Choose Anti-Inflammatory Foods: Opt for menu items rich in anti-inflammatory ingredients. Fatty fish, leafy greens, nuts, and berries are not only delicious but can also contribute to managing inflammation.

➢ Inquire About Cooking Preparation:s: Ask about how dishes are prepared. Grilled, baked, or steamed options are often preferable to fried or heavily sautéed choices. These cooking Preparation:s retain nutritional value without excess saturated fats.

➢ Customize Your Order: Don't hesitate to customize your meal based on your dietary preferences and restrictions. Restaurants are often willing to accommodate special requests regarding ingredients or cooking methods.

➢ Prioritize Omega-3s: Include omega-3 fatty acids in your meal. Salmon or other fatty fish can provide joint-friendly nutrients that may help alleviate symptoms associated with RA.

➢ Ask for Sauce on the Side: Requesting sauces and dressings on the side gives you control over how much you add to your meal. This allows for a flavorful experience without overwhelming your taste buds or potentially causing discomfort.

➢ Opt for Whole Grains: When possible, choose whole grains over refined carbohydrates. Quinoa, brown rice, or whole wheat options provide more nutrients and may contribute to a more balanced meal.

➢ Stay Hydrated: Adequate hydration is essential, especially when dining out. Water not only supports overall health but also helps manage potential side effects of RA medications.

➢ Choose Comfortable Seating: Select a restaurant with comfortable seating and ample space. Cushioned chairs and adequate room to move can enhance comfort during your dining experience.

➢ Inform Waitstaff About Dietary Needs: If you have specific dietary needs or allergies, communicate them to the waitstaff. This ensures that your meal is prepared according to your requirements.

➢ Mindful Eating Practices: Eat slowly, savoring each bite. Mindful eating not only enhances the dining experience but also promotes awareness of hunger and fullness cues, preventing overeating.

By adopting these dining-out strategies, individuals with RA can make choices that support their overall well-being while still relishing the pleasure of a restaurant meal. Taking a proactive approach to dining out empowers individuals to enjoy social occasions without compromising their health goals or exacerbating RA symptoms.

The art of cooking extends beyond creating delicious meals; it involves preserving the nutritional value and flavors of ingredients. Employing certain cooking techniques ensures that the dishes not only tantalize the taste buds but also retain essential nutrients. Here are some cooking strategies to preserve both the goodness and the richness of flavors:

➤ Steaming: Steaming is a gentle cooking method that minimizes nutrient loss. Vegetables, fish, and even grains can be steamed to preserve vitamins and minerals. This technique also helps maintain the natural color and texture of the ingredients.

➤ Sautéing: Quick sautéing in a small amount of oil over high heat is an effective way to lock in flavors while maintaining the nutritional integrity of vegetables and lean proteins. It's important to avoid overcooking to prevent nutrient degradation.

➤ Grilling: Grilling imparts a smoky flavor to food while allowing excess fat to drip away. This technique is ideal for meats, vegetables, and even fruits. To preserve nutrients, marinate items before grilling and avoid prolonged cooking times.

➤ Blanching: Blanching involves briefly immersing vegetables in boiling water, followed by rapid cooling. This Preparation: helps retain color, flavor, and nutrients. It is particularly effective for vegetables like broccoli and green beans.

➤ Roasting: Roasting vegetables and certain meats enhances their natural flavors.

➢ Use minimal oil, and keep an eye on cooking times to prevent nutrient loss. Roasting at lower temperatures for a longer duration is preferable for nutrient preservation.

➢ Poaching: Poaching involves cooking food in a simmering liquid. This gentle method is suitable for delicate proteins like fish and eggs. Poaching helps retain moisture and prevents the leaching of nutrients.

➢ Raw Preparations: Embracing raw preparations, such as salads and smoothies, allows you to enjoy ingredients in their natural state. Raw foods often contain higher levels of certain nutrients that can be sensitive to heat.

➢ Microwaving: While often underestimated, microwaving is a quick and efficient cooking Preparation: that can help preserve nutrients. Short cooking times and minimal use of water contribute to nutrient retention.

➢ Use of Herbs and Spices: Enhance flavor without relying on excessive salt or sugar by incorporating a variety of herbs and spices. These additions not only elevate taste but also contribute antioxidants and other health-promoting compounds.

By employing these cooking techniques, individuals can create meals that are not only delicious but also nutritionally robust. Balancing flavor and nutrient preservation allows for a culinary experience that not only satisfies the palate but also nourishes the body.

CHAPTER SIX: Rheumatoid Arthritis Recipes

BREAKFAST RECIPES:

1. Golden Turmeric Smoothie:

Ingredients:

- 1 cup unsweetened almond milk
- 1/2 banana
- 1/2 teaspoon turmeric powder
- 1/4 teaspoon ginger
- 1 tablespoon chia seeds

Preparation:

- Blend all ingredients until smooth.

Health Benefits:

- Turmeric and ginger have anti-inflammatory properties.

Cooking Time: 5 minutes

2. Quinoa Breakfast Bowl:

Ingredients:

- Cooked quinoa
- Fresh berries
- Nuts (almonds or walnuts)
- Greek yogurt
- Honey

Preparation:

> Mix quinoa with berries, nuts, and top with Greek yogurt. Drizzle honey.

Health Benefits:

> Quinoa is a protein-rich grain with essential amino acids.

Cooking Time: 15 minutes (if quinoa is pre-cooked)

3. Avocado and Smoked Salmon Toast:

Ingredients:

> Whole-grain bread
> Ripe avocado
> Smoked salmon
> Lemon juice
> Dill

Preparation:

> Toast bread, spread mashed avocado, top with smoked salmon, a squeeze of lemon, and dill.

Health Benefits:

> Avocado provides healthy fats; salmon is rich in omega-3 fatty acids.

Cooking Time: 10 minutes

4. Berry and Spinach Smoothie Bowl:

Ingredients:

- Mixed berries (frozen or fresh)
- Spinach leaves
- Greek yogurt
- Almond milk
- Granola and seeds for topping

Preparation:

- Blend berries, spinach, yogurt, and almond milk. Top with granola and seeds.

Health Benefits:

- Berries and spinach offer antioxidants and vitamins.

Cooking Time: 5 minutes

5. Oatmeal with Almond Butter and Banana:

Ingredients:

- Rolled oats
- Almond butter
- Banana slices
- Cinnamon
- Honey (optional)

Preparation:

> ➢ Cook oats, top with almond butter, banana slices, a sprinkle of cinnamon, and honey if desired.

Health Benefits:

> ➢ Oats are a good source of fiber; almond butter provides healthy fats.

Cooking Time: 10 minutes

6. Veggie Omelette with Turmeric:

Ingredients:

> ➢ Eggs
> ➢ Mixed vegetables (bell peppers, spinach, tomatoes)
> ➢ Turmeric powder
> ➢ Olive oil

Preparation:

> ➢ Sauté vegetables, add beaten eggs with turmeric. Cook until set.

Health Benefits:

> ➢ Turmeric has anti-inflammatory properties; veggies add vitamins.

Cooking Time: 15 minutes

7. Chia Seed Pudding with Berries:

Ingredients:

- ➤ Chia seeds
- ➤ Almond milk
- ➤ Mixed berries
- ➤ Maple syrup

Preparation:

- ➤ Mix chia seeds with almond milk, refrigerate overnight. Top with berries and a drizzle of maple syrup.

Health Benefits:

- ➤ Chia seeds are rich in omega-3 fatty acids.

Cooking Time: Overnight, plus 5 minutes

8. Spinach and Mushroom Breakfast Wrap:

Ingredients:

Whole-grain wrap

Eggs

Spinach

Mushrooms

Feta cheese

Preparation:

> Sauté spinach and mushrooms, scramble eggs, fill the wrap, and top with feta.

Health Benefits:

> Spinach and mushrooms provide vitamins and minerals.

Cooking Time: 10 minutes

9. Apple Cinnamon Overnight Oats:

Ingredients:

> Rolled oats
> Greek yogurt
> Almond milk
> Chopped apples
> Cinnamon

Preparation:

> Mix oats, yogurt, almond milk, apples, and cinnamon. Refrigerate overnight.

Health Benefits:

> Oats and apples contribute fiber and antioxidants.

Cooking Time: Overnight

10. Sweet Potato and Kale Breakfast Hash:

Ingredients:

- Sweet potatoes, diced
- Kale, chopped
- Red onion, diced
- Eggs
- Olive oil

Preparation:

- Sauté sweet potatoes, kale, and onions. Add eggs and cook until desired doneness.

Health Benefits:

- Sweet potatoes and kale are rich in vitamins and minerals.

Cooking Time: 20 minutes

LUNCH RECIPES:

1. Quinoa and Chickpea Salad:

Ingredients:

- Cooked quinoa
- Canned chickpeas, drained and rinsed
- Cherry tomatoes, halved
- Cucumber, diced
- Red onion, finely chopped
- Feta cheese, crumbled

➢ Olive oil, lemon juice, garlic, oregano

Preparation:

➢ Combine quinoa, chickpeas, tomatoes, cucumber, red onion, and feta in a bowl.

➢ Mix olive oil, lemon juice, minced garlic, and oregano for dressing.

➢ Pour dressing over the salad, toss, and serve.

Health Benefits:

➢ Rich in protein, fiber, and anti-inflammatory ingredients.

Cooking Time: 15 minutes.

2. Salmon and Sweet Potato Foil Packets:

Ingredients:

➢ Salmon fillets

➢ Sweet potatoes, thinly sliced

➢ Asparagus spears

➢ Lemon slices

➢ Olive oil, garlic, dill

Preparation:

➢ Place salmon on foil, surround with sweet potatoes and asparagus.

➢ Drizzle with olive oil, minced garlic, and dill.

➢ Seal packets and bake until salmon is cooked.

Health Benefits:

> ➤ Omega-3 fatty acids, anti-inflammatory compounds.

Cooking Time: 20 minutes.

3. Turkey and Vegetable Stir-Fry:

Ingredients:

> ➤ Ground turkey
> ➤ Mixed vegetables (bell peppers, broccoli, snap peas)
> ➤ Low-sodium soy sauce, ginger, garlic
> ➤ Brown rice or quinoa

Preparation:

> ➤ Stir-fry ground turkey and vegetables in a wok.
> ➤ Add soy sauce, minced ginger, and garlic.
> ➤ Serve over cooked brown rice or quinoa.

Health Benefits:

> ➤ Lean protein, antioxidants, anti-inflammatory properties.

Cooking Time: 15 minutes.

4. Greek Chicken Wrap:

Ingredients:

> ➤ Grilled chicken strips
> ➤ Whole wheat wrap
> ➤ Greek yogurt

- ➢ Cucumber, tomatoes, red onion
- ➢ Feta cheese, olives

Preparation:

- ➢ Assemble grilled chicken, veggies, and feta in a wrap.
- ➢ Drizzle with Greek yogurt.

Health Benefits:

- ➢ Protein, whole grains, calcium.

Cooking Time: 10 minutes.

5. Lentil and Vegetable Soup:

Ingredients:

- ➢ Brown lentils
- ➢ Carrots, celery, onions
- ➢ Vegetable broth, tomatoes
- ➢ Garlic, cumin, coriander

Preparation:

- ➢ Sauté veggies, add lentils, broth, and spices.
- ➢ Simmer until lentils are tender.

Health Benefits:

- ➢ Fiber, plant-based protein, anti-inflammatory spices.

Cooking Time: 30 minutes.

6. Spinach and Walnut Salad with Grilled Chicken:

Ingredients:

- ➢ Grilled chicken breast
- ➢ Fresh spinach leaves
- ➢ Cherry tomatoes, avocado
- ➢ Walnuts, feta cheese
- ➢ Balsamic vinaigrette

Preparation:

- ➢ Combine grilled chicken, spinach, tomatoes, avocado, walnuts, and feta.
- ➢ Drizzle with balsamic vinaigrette.

Health Benefits:

- ➢ Omega-3 fatty acids, antioxidants, vitamin K.

Cooking Time: 15 minutes.

7. Veggie and Quinoa Stuffed Peppers:

Ingredients:

- ➢ Quinoa, cooked
- ➢ Bell peppers, halved
- ➢ Black beans, corn, tomatoes
- ➢ Chili powder, cumin

Preparation:

> Mix quinoa with black beans, corn, tomatoes, and spices.

> Stuff the pepper halves and bake until tender.

Health Benefits:

> Protein, fiber, vitamin C.

Cooking Time: 25 minutes.

8. Tofu and Vegetable Curry:

Ingredients:

> Extra-firm tofu

> Mixed vegetables (bell peppers, broccoli, carrots)

> Coconut milk, curry paste

> Brown rice

Preparation:

> Sauté tofu and veggies, add coconut milk and curry paste.

> Simmer until vegetables are tender.

Health Benefits:

> Plant-based protein, antioxidants.

Cooking Time: 20 minutes.

9. Avocado and Black Bean Wrap:

Ingredients:

- Black beans, canned and rinsed
- Avocado, mashed
- Whole wheat wrap
- Salsa, lettuce, cheese

Preparation:

- Mix black beans with mashed avocado.
- Spread the mixture on a wrap, add salsa, lettuce, and cheese.

Health Benefits:

- Healthy fats, fiber, plant-based protein.

Cooking Time: 10 minutes.

10. Egg and Vegetable Fried Rice:

Ingredients:

- Brown rice, cooked
- Eggs, beaten
- Mixed vegetables (peas, carrots, corn)
- Soy sauce, sesame oil

Preparation:

- Stir-fry veggies, add cooked rice and eggs.
- Season with soy sauce and sesame oil.

Health Benefits:

- ➢ Protein, fiber, essential amino acids.

Cooking Time: 15 minutes.

DINNER RECIPES:

1. Grilled Salmon with Quinoa and Roasted Vegetables:

Ingredients:

- ➢ Salmon fillets
- ➢ Quinoa
- ➢ Assorted vegetables (bell peppers, zucchini, cherry tomatoes)
- ➢ Olive oil, lemon, herbs

Preparation:

- ➢ Marinate salmon in olive oil, lemon juice, and herbs.
- ➢ Grill salmon while roasting vegetables.
- ➢ Cook quinoa according to package instructions.
- ➢ Serve grilled salmon on a bed of quinoa with roasted vegetables.

Health Benefits:

- ➢ Omega-3 fatty acids in salmon reduce inflammation.
- ➢ Quinoa provides protein and essential amino acids.
- ➢ Vegetables offer antioxidants and fiber.

Cooking Time: 25 minutes

2. Lentil and Vegetable Curry:

Ingredients:

- ➢ Lentils
- ➢ Mixed vegetables (carrots, spinach, bell peppers)
- ➢ Coconut milk, curry spices, garlic, ginger
- ➢ Brown rice

Preparation:

- ➢ Cook lentils and vegetables in coconut milk with curry spices, garlic, and ginger.
- ➢ Serve over cooked brown rice.

Health Benefits:

- ➢ Lentils are rich in protein and fiber.
- ➢ Vegetables provide vitamins and antioxidants.
- ➢ Coconut milk adds healthy fats.

Cooking Time: 30 minutes

3. Quinoa and Chickpea Stuffed Bell Peppers:

Ingredients:

- ➢ Bell peppers
- ➢ Quinoa
- ➢ Chickpeas, tomatoes, onions, garlic
- ➢ Spices, herbs

Preparation:

> ➢ Cook quinoa and sauté chickpeas, tomatoes, onions, and garlic with spices.
> ➢ Stuff bell peppers with the quinoa-chickpea mixture.
> ➢ Bake until peppers are tender.

Health Benefits:

> ➢ Quinoa offers protein and essential nutrients.
> ➢ Chickpeas provide protein and fiber.
> ➢ Bell peppers are rich in vitamin C.

Cooking Time: 40 minutes

4. Baked Cod with Herbed Quinoa and Steamed Broccoli:

Ingredients:

> ➢ Cod fillets
> ➢ Quinoa
> ➢ Fresh herbs (parsley, dill)
> ➢ Broccoli
> ➢ Lemon, olive oil, garlic

Preparation:

> ➢ Season cod with herbs, lemon, and olive oil, then bake.
> ➢ Cook quinoa with garlic and herbs.
> ➢ Steam broccoli until tender.
> ➢ Serve cod over herbed quinoa with steamed broccoli.

Health Benefits:

- ➢ Cod is a lean protein source.
- ➢ Quinoa provides essential amino acids.
- ➢ Broccoli is rich in antioxidants.

Cooking Time: 30 minutes

5. Spinach and Mushroom Stuffed Chicken Breast:

Ingredients:

- ➢ Chicken breasts
- ➢ Spinach, mushrooms, feta cheese
- ➢ Olive oil, garlic, herbs

Preparation:

- ➢ Sauté spinach, mushrooms, and garlic, then mix with feta.
- ➢ Cut a pocket in chicken breasts and stuff with the spinach mixture.
- ➢ Season with herbs and bake until chicken is cooked through.

Health Benefits:

- ➢ Chicken is a lean protein source.
- ➢ Spinach and mushrooms offer vitamins and minerals.
- ➢ Feta adds a burst of flavor.

Cooking Time: 35 minutes

6. Vegetable Stir-Fry with Tofu:

Ingredients:

- Tofu
- Mixed vegetables (broccoli, bell peppers, snap peas)
- Soy sauce, ginger, garlic
- Brown rice or quinoa

Preparation:

- Stir-fry tofu and mixed vegetables in a wok with soy sauce, ginger, and garlic.
- Serve over cooked brown rice or quinoa.

Health Benefits:

- Tofu provides plant-based protein.
- Mixed vegetables offer fiber and antioxidants.
- Soy sauce adds flavor without excess salt.

Cooking Time: 25 minutes

7. Turkey and Sweet Potato Chili:

Ingredients:

- Ground turkey
- Sweet potatoes, black beans, diced tomatoes
- Chili spices, garlic, onion

Preparation:

> Brown turkey with garlic and onion.
> Add sweet potatoes, black beans, diced tomatoes, and chili spices.
> Simmer until sweet potatoes are tender.

Health Benefits:

> Turkey is a lean protein source.
> Sweet potatoes provide vitamins and fiber.
> Black beans offer protein and antioxidants.

Cooking Time: 40 minutes

8. Shrimp and Quinoa Paella:

Ingredients:

> Shrimp
> Quinoa
> Bell peppers, tomatoes, peas
> Saffron, paprika, garlic

Preparation:

> Sauté shrimp with garlic, then add bell peppers, tomatoes, and peas.
> Stir in quinoa, saffron, and paprika.
> Cook until quinoa is done.

Health Benefits:

- ➤ Shrimp provides lean protein.
- ➤ Quinoa offers essential amino acids.
- ➤ Bell peppers and tomatoes add vitamins.

Cooking Time: 35 minutes

9. Mediterranean Eggplant and Chickpea Bake:

Ingredients:

- ➤ Eggplant
- ➤ Chickpeas
- ➤ Tomatoes, red onion, garlic
- ➤ Olive oil, oregano, feta cheese

Preparation:

- ➤ Layer sliced eggplant, chickpeas, tomatoes, red onion, and garlic in a baking dish.
- ➤ Drizzle with olive oil, sprinkle with oregano, and bake until vegetables are tender.
- ➤ Top with crumbled feta before serving.

Health Benefits:

- ➤ Eggplant provides fiber and antioxidants.
- ➤ Chickpeas offer protein and fiber.
- ➤ Tomatoes and red onion add vitamins.

Cooking Time: 45 minutes

10. Butternut Squash and Lentil Stew:

Ingredients:

- ➤ Butternut squash
- ➤ Lentils
- ➤ Carrots, celery, onion
- ➤ Vegetable broth, spices

Preparation:

- ➤ Sauté carrots, celery, and onion until softened.
- ➤ Add butternut squash, lentils, vegetable broth, and spices.
- ➤ Simmer until vegetables and lentils are tender.

Health Benefits:

- ➤ Butternut squash is rich in vitamins A and C.
- ➤ Lentils provide protein and fiber.
- ➤ Carrots and celery add vitamins and crunch.

Cooking Time: 50 minutes

SNACK RECIPES:

1. Nutty Yogurt Parfait:

Ingredients:

- ➤ Greek yogurt
- ➤ Mixed nuts (almonds, walnuts, pistachios)
- ➤ Honey

Preparation:

- Layer Greek yogurt with mixed nuts in a glass.
- Drizzle honey over the top.

Health Benefits:

- Rich in protein and healthy fats.
- Provides essential nutrients like calcium and antioxidants.

Cooking Time: 5 minutes

2. Roasted Chickpeas:

Ingredients:

- Canned chickpeas, drained
- Olive oil
- Paprika, cumin, garlic powder

Preparation:

- Toss chickpeas in olive oil and spices.
- Roast in the oven until crispy.
- Health Benefits:
- High in protein and fiber.
- Supports joint health.

Cooking Time: 20 minutes

3. Veggie Sticks with Hummus:

Ingredients:

- ➢ Carrot and cucumber sticks
- ➢ Hummus
- ➢ Preparation:
- ➢ Arrange vegetable sticks on a plate.
- ➢ Serve with a side of hummus.

Health Benefits:

- ➢ Provides vitamins, fiber, and healthy fats.
- ➢ Hummus offers protein and anti-inflammatory properties.

Cooking Time: 5 minutes

4. Turmeric and Ginger Tea:

Ingredients:

- ➢ Fresh turmeric
- ➢ Fresh ginger
- ➢ Honey

Preparation:

- ➢ Grate turmeric and ginger into hot water.
- ➢ Sweeten with honey.

Health Benefits:

- ➢ Anti-inflammatory properties of turmeric and ginger.

➢ Soothes joint pain.

Cooking Time: 10 minutes

5. Berry Smoothie Bowl:

Ingredients:

➢ Mixed berries (strawberries, blueberries, raspberries)

➢ Greek yogurt

➢ Chia seeds

Preparation:

➢ Blend berries with Greek yogurt.

➢ Pour into a bowl and top with chia seeds.

Health Benefits:

➢ Rich in antioxidants and vitamins.

➢ Greek yogurt adds protein.

Cooking Time: 5 minutes

6. Almond and Date Energy Bites:

Ingredients:

➢ Almonds

➢ Dates

➢ Coconut flakes

Preparation:

➢ Blend almonds and dates in a food processor.

> Roll into bite-sized balls and coat with coconut flakes.

Health Benefits:

> Provides energy and essential nutrients.
> Almonds contain anti-inflammatory properties.

Cooking Time: 15 minutes

7. Avocado Toast with Tomato:

Ingredients:

> Whole-grain bread
> Avocado
> Tomato slices

Preparation:

> Toast bread and spread mashed avocado.
> Top with tomato slices.

Health Benefits:

> Healthy fats in avocado.
> Tomatoes contain antioxidants.

Cooking Time: 5 minutes

8. Quinoa Salad Cups:

Ingredients:

> Cooked quinoa
> Cucumber, cherry tomatoes, feta cheese

➤ Olive oil, lemon juice, herbs

Preparation:

➤ Mix quinoa with chopped vegetables and feta.

➤ Drizzle with olive oil, lemon juice, and herbs.

Health Benefits:

➤ Quinoa provides protein and fiber.

➤ Vegetables offer antioxidants and vitamins.

Cooking Time: 15 minutes

9. Spinach and Artichoke Dip:

Ingredients:

➤ Frozen spinach, thawed

➤ Artichoke hearts, chopped

➤ Greek yogurt, cream cheese

Preparation:

➤ Mix ingredients and bake until bubbly.

➤ Health Benefits:

➤ Spinach is rich in iron and antioxidants.

➤ Greek yogurt adds protein.

Cooking Time: 20 minutes

10. Dark Chocolate and Almond Clusters:

Ingredients:

- Dark chocolate
- Almonds
- Sea salt

Preparation:

- Melt dark chocolate and mix with almonds.
- Drop clusters onto a parchment-lined tray, sprinkle with sea salt, and refrigerate.

Health Benefits:

- Dark chocolate contains antioxidants.
- Almonds provide healthy fats and vitamin E.

Cooking Time: 10 minutes

SOUP RECIPES:

1. Turmeric Ginger Carrot Soup:

Ingredients:

- Carrots, peeled and chopped
- Fresh ginger, grated
- Turmeric powder
- Vegetable broth
- Coconut milk
- Onion, diced

Preparation:

- ➢ Sauté onions and ginger in a pot until softened.
- ➢ Add carrots, turmeric, and vegetable broth.
- ➢ Simmer until carrots are tender, then blend until smooth.
- ➢ Stir in coconut milk and heat through.

Health Benefits:

- ➢ Anti-inflammatory properties of turmeric and ginger.
- ➢ Beta-carotene from carrots supports immune function.

Cooking Time: 30 minutes

2. Quinoa and Kale Soup:

Ingredients:

- ➢ Quinoa
- ➢ Kale, chopped
- ➢ Vegetable broth
- ➢ Garlic, minced
- ➢ Cannellini beans, drained
- ➢ Tomatoes, diced

Preparation:

- ➢ Cook quinoa separately.
- ➢ Sauté garlic, add kale, beans, and tomatoes.
- ➢ Pour in vegetable broth and cooked quinoa.
- ➢ Simmer until kale is tender.

Health Benefits:

- ➢ Quinoa provides protein and fiber.
- ➢ Kale is rich in vitamins and antioxidants.

Cooking Time: 25 minutes

3. Lentil and Spinach Soup:

Ingredients:

- ➢ Lentils, rinsed
- ➢ Spinach, chopped
- ➢ Onion, diced
- ➢ Cumin, coriander, turmeric
- ➢ Vegetable broth
- ➢ Lemon juice

Preparation:

- ➢ Sauté onions and spices until fragrant.
- ➢ Add lentils, vegetable broth, and simmer.
- ➢ Stir in spinach and cook until wilted.
- ➢ Finish with a squeeze of lemon juice.

Health Benefits:

- ➢ Lentils offer protein and iron.
- ➢ Spinach provides vitamins and minerals.

Cooking Time: 35 minutes

4. Sweet Potato and Coconut Soup:

Ingredients:

- Sweet potatoes, peeled and cubed
- Coconut milk
- Ginger, grated
- Vegetable broth
- Red curry paste
- Garlic, minced

Preparation:

- Sauté garlic and ginger, add red curry paste.
- Add sweet potatoes, coconut milk, and vegetable broth.
- Simmer until sweet potatoes are tender.
- Blend until smooth.

Health Benefits:

- Sweet potatoes are rich in antioxidants and anti-inflammatory compounds.
- Coconut milk provides healthy fats.

Cooking Time: 40 minutes

5. Broccoli and Almond Soup:

Ingredients:

- Broccoli, chopped
- Almonds, toasted

➢ Onion, diced

➢ Vegetable broth

➢ Nutmeg

➢ Greek yogurt (optional)

Preparation:

➢ Sauté onions until translucent, add broccoli.

➢ Pour in vegetable broth and simmer.

➢ Blend with toasted almonds until smooth.

➢ Season with nutmeg, and add a dollop of Greek yogurt if desired.

Health Benefits:

➢ Broccoli is rich in vitamins K and C.

➢ Almonds provide healthy fats and vitamin E.

Cooking Time: 30 minutes

6. Butternut Squash and Apple Soup:

Ingredients:

➢ Butternut squash, peeled and cubed

➢ Apples, peeled and chopped

➢ Onion, diced

➢ Vegetable broth

➢ Cinnamon, nutmeg

➢ Coconut oil

Preparation:

- ➢ Sauté onions in coconut oil, add squash and apples.
- ➢ Pour in vegetable broth and simmer.
- ➢ Blend until smooth, season with cinnamon and nutmeg.

Health Benefits:

- ➢ Butternut squash is rich in vitamin A and potassium.
- ➢ Apples add natural sweetness and fiber.

Cooking Time: 35 minutes

7. Red Lentil and Tomato Soup:

Ingredients:

- ➢ Red lentils, rinsed
- ➢ Tomatoes, diced
- ➢ Carrots, chopped
- ➢ Garlic, minced
- ➢ Cumin, paprika
- ➢ Vegetable broth

Preparation:

- ➢ Sauté garlic, add cumin and paprika.
- ➢ Stir in lentils, tomatoes, and carrots.
- ➢ Pour in vegetable broth and simmer until lentils are cooked.
- ➢ Blend to desired consistency.

Health Benefits:

- ➢ Red lentils are a good source of protein and iron.
- ➢ Tomatoes provide antioxidants like lycopene.

Cooking Time: 25 minutes

8. Spicy Chicken and Vegetable Soup:

Ingredients:

- ➢ Chicken breast, cooked and shredded
- ➢ Bell peppers, diced
- ➢ Jalapeños, sliced
- ➢ Corn, kernels
- ➢ Chicken broth
- ➢ Cumin, chili powder, lime juice

Preparation:

- ➢ Sauté bell peppers and jalapeños, add shredded chicken.
- ➢ Pour in chicken broth, add corn.
- ➢ Season with cumin, chili powder, and lime juice.
- ➢ Simmer until flavors meld.

Health Benefits:

- ➢ Chicken provides lean protein.
- ➢ Bell peppers offer vitamin C and antioxidants.

Cooking Time: 30 minutes

9. Cauliflower and Leek Soup:

Ingredients:

- Cauliflower, chopped
- Leeks, sliced
- Garlic, minced
- Vegetable broth
- Thyme, bay leaves
- Olive oil

Preparation:

- Sauté leeks and garlic in olive oil.
- Add cauliflower, vegetable broth, thyme, and bay leaves.
- Simmer until cauliflower is tender.
- Remove bay leaves and blend until smooth.

Health Benefits:

- Cauliflower is rich in vitamins C and K.
- Leeks provide a mild onion flavor and fiber.

Cooking Time: 35 minutes

10. Black Bean and Spinach Soup:

Ingredients:

- Black beans, canned and rinsed
- Spinach, chopped
- Tomatoes, diced

- ➢ Cumin, coriander, garlic powder
- ➢ Vegetable broth
- ➢ Lime juice

Preparation:

- ➢ Combine black beans, tomatoes, and spinach in a pot.
- ➢ Add vegetable broth, cumin, coriander, and garlic powder.
- ➢ Simmer until flavors meld.
- ➢ Finish with a squeeze of lime juice.

Health Benefits:

- ➢ Black beans offer protein and fiber.
- ➢ Spinach provides iron and vitamins A and C.

Cooking Time: 25 minutes

BONE HEALTH RECIPES:

1. Calcium-Rich Green Smoothie:

Ingredients:

- ➢ Kale or spinach
- ➢ Greek yogurt
- ➢ Banana
- ➢ Almond milk
- ➢ Chia seeds

Preparation: Preparation:

> Blend kale/spinach, Greek yogurt, banana, almond milk, and chia seeds until smooth.

Health Benefits:

> High in calcium from yogurt and leafy greens.
> Provides vitamin K and magnesium for bone health.

Cooking Time: 5 minutes

2. Salmon and Quinoa Salad:

Ingredients:

> Grilled salmon
> Quinoa
> Mixed greens
> Cherry tomatoes
> Avocado
> Lemon-tahini dressing

Preparation:

> Combine grilled salmon, cooked quinoa, mixed greens, cherry tomatoes, and avocado.
> Drizzle with lemon-tahini dressing.

Health Benefits:

> Omega-3 fatty acids from salmon.
> Quinoa offers calcium and magnesium.

Cooking Time: 20 minutes

3. Turmeric-Ginger Lentil Soup:

Ingredients:

- ➢ Red lentils
- ➢ Turmeric
- ➢ Ginger
- ➢ Carrots
- ➢ Celery
- ➢ Vegetable broth

Preparation:

- ➢ Sauté onions, carrots, and celery with turmeric and ginger.
- ➢ Add red lentils and vegetable broth, simmer until lentils are tender.

Health Benefits:

- ➢ Turmeric and ginger have anti-inflammatory properties.
- ➢ Lentils provide protein and iron.

Cooking Time: 30 minutes

4. Grilled Veggie Skewers with Tofu:

Ingredients:

- ➢ Bell peppers
- ➢ Zucchini
- ➢ Cherry tomatoes

- ➢ Firm tofu
- ➢ Olive oil, garlic, herbs

Preparation:

- ➢ Thread veggies and tofu onto skewers.
- ➢ Brush with olive oil, garlic, and herbs before grilling.

Health Benefits:

- ➢ Tofu offers plant-based protein.
- ➢ Veggies provide vitamins and minerals.

Cooking Time: 15 minutes

5. Quinoa-Stuffed Acorn Squash:

Ingredients:

- ➢ Acorn squash
- ➢ Quinoa
- ➢ Spinach
- ➢ Pecans
- ➢ Cranberries

Preparation:

- ➢ Roast acorn squash halves.
- ➢ Fill with a mixture of cooked quinoa, sautéed spinach, pecans, and cranberries.

Health Benefits:

> Quinoa is a complete protein.
> Spinach offers iron and vitamin K.

Cooking Time: 40 minutes

6. Greek Yogurt Parfait with Berries:

Ingredients:

> Greek yogurt
> Mixed berries (blueberries, strawberries)
> Almonds
> Honey

Preparation:

> Layer Greek yogurt with mixed berries and almonds.
> Drizzle with honey.

Health Benefits:

> Greek yogurt provides calcium and protein.
> Berries offer antioxidants.

Cooking Time: 5 minutes

7. Walnut-Crusted Baked Chicken:

Ingredients:

> Chicken breasts
> Walnuts

- ➢ Dijon mustard

- ➢ Herbs (rosemary, thyme)

Preparation:

- ➢ Coat chicken with a mixture of crushed walnuts, Dijon mustard, and herbs.

- ➢ Bake until chicken is cooked through.

Health Benefits:

- ➢ Walnuts contain omega-3 fatty acids.

- ➢ Chicken provides lean protein.

Cooking Time: 25 minutes

8. Spinach and Feta Stuffed Mushrooms:

Ingredients:

- ➢ Portobello mushrooms

- ➢ Spinach

- ➢ Feta cheese

- ➢ Garlic

- ➢ Olive oil

Preparation: Preparation:

- ➢ Sauté spinach and garlic, mix with feta.

- ➢ Stuff mushrooms, drizzle with olive oil, and bake.

Health Benefits:

> Spinach is rich in vitamin K.
> Feta provides calcium.

Cooking Time: 20 minutes

9. Avocado and Black Bean Salad:

Ingredients:

> Black beans (canned)
> Avocado
> Corn
> Red onion
> Cilantro

Preparation:

> Combine black beans, diced avocado, corn, red onion, and cilantro.
> Toss with olive oil and lime juice.

Health Benefits:

> Black beans offer protein and fiber.
> Avocado provides healthy fats.

Cooking Time: 10 minutes

10. Sweet Potato and Chickpea Curry:

Ingredients:

- ➢ Sweet potatoes
- ➢ Chickpeas
- ➢ Coconut milk
- ➢ Curry spices
- ➢ Spinach

Preparation:

- ➢ Sauté sweet potatoes, chickpeas, and curry spices.
- ➢ Add coconut milk and simmer until sweet potatoes are tender.
- ➢ Stir in spinach until wilted.

Health Benefits:

- ➢ Sweet potatoes are rich in vitamin A.
- ➢ Chickpeas offer protein and fiber.

Cooking Time: 30 minutes

ANTI-INFLAMMATORY RECIPES:

1. Turmeric-Ginger Golden Milk:

Ingredients:

- ➢ 1 cup almond milk
- ➢ 1 teaspoon turmeric powder
- ➢ 1/2 teaspoon ginger powder
- ➢ 1 tablespoon honey

Preparation:

> Heat almond milk, turmeric, and ginger in a saucepan.

> Simmer for 5 minutes, stirring occasionally.

> Add honey and mix well before serving.

Health Benefits:

> Turmeric and ginger have anti-inflammatory properties that may help alleviate RA symptoms.

Cooking Time: 10 minutes

2. Quinoa and Vegetable Buddha Bowl:

Ingredients:

> Cooked quinoa

> Mixed vegetables (broccoli, bell peppers, carrots)

> Avocado slices

> Olive oil and lemon dressing

Preparation:

> Roast or sauté vegetables until tender.

> Arrange quinoa, vegetables, and avocado in a bowl.

> Drizzle with olive oil and lemon dressing.

Health Benefits:

> Quinoa is a protein-rich grain, and vegetables provide antioxidants for anti-inflammatory effects.

Cooking Time: 20 minutes

3. Salmon and Kale Salad:

Ingredients:

- ➤ Grilled salmon fillet
- ➤ Fresh kale, chopped
- ➤ Cherry tomatoes, halved
- ➤ Lemon-tahini dressing

Preparation:

- ➤ Grill salmon until cooked.
- ➤ Toss kale and cherry tomatoes in a bowl.
- ➤ Top with grilled salmon and drizzle with lemon-tahini dressing.

Health Benefits:

- ➤ Omega-3 fatty acids in salmon contribute to anti-inflammatory effects.

Cooking Time: 15 minutes

4. Chickpea and Spinach Stew:

Ingredients:

- ➤ Canned chickpeas, drained
- ➤ Fresh spinach
- ➤ Tomatoes, diced
- ➤ Garlic, minced
- ➤ Cumin and coriander for seasoning

Preparation:

- ➤ Sauté garlic in olive oil.
- ➤ Add chickpeas, tomatoes, and spices.
- ➤ Stir in fresh spinach and simmer until wilted.

Health Benefits:

- ➤ Chickpeas are rich in fiber and anti-inflammatory compounds.

Cooking Time: 20 minutes

5. Mediterranean Lentil Soup:

Ingredients:

- ➤ Lentils
- ➤ Carrots, celery, onions
- ➤ Garlic, minced
- ➤ Vegetable broth
- ➤ Mediterranean herbs (rosemary, thyme)

Preparation:

- ➤ Sauté garlic, carrots, celery, and onions.
- ➤ Add lentils, vegetable broth, and herbs.
- ➤ Simmer until lentils are tender.

Health Benefits:

- ➤ Lentils provide protein and fiber with anti-inflammatory properties.

Cooking Time: 30 minutes

6. Spinach and Berry Smoothie:

Ingredients:

- Fresh spinach
- Mixed berries (blueberries, strawberries)
- Greek yogurt
- Almond milk

Preparation:

- Blend spinach, berries, Greek yogurt, and almond milk until smooth.
- Optional: Add a teaspoon of chia seeds.

Health Benefits:

- Berries are rich in antioxidants with potential anti-inflammatory effects.

Cooking Time: 5 minutes

7. Walnut and Kale Pesto Pasta:

Ingredients:

- Whole-grain pasta
- Kale, blanched
- Walnuts
- Parmesan cheese
- Olive oil

Preparation:

> Blend kale, walnuts, Parmesan, and olive oil into a pesto sauce.

> Toss with cooked whole-grain pasta.

Health Benefits:

> Walnuts provide omega-3 fatty acids for anti-inflammatory benefits.

Cooking Time: 15 minutes

8. Cauliflower and Chickpea Curry:

Ingredients:

> Cauliflower, chopped

> Chickpeas, cooked

> Coconut milk

> Curry spices (turmeric, cumin, coriander)

Preparation:

> Sauté cauliflower in curry spices.

> Add cooked chickpeas and coconut milk.

> Simmer until cauliflower is tender.

Health Benefits:

> Turmeric in curry spices has potent anti-inflammatory properties.

Cooking Time: 25 minutes

9. Avocado and Black Bean Salad:

Ingredients:

- Black beans, canned
- Avocado, diced
- Red onion, finely chopped
- Cilantro, chopped
- Lime vinaigrette

Preparation:

- Combine black beans, avocado, red onion, and cilantro.
- Toss with lime vinaigrette before serving.

Health Benefits:

- Avocado provides healthy fats with anti-inflammatory effects.

Cooking Time: 10 minutes

10. Berry and Almond Chia Pudding:

Ingredients:

- Chia seeds
- Almond milk
- Mixed berries
- Almonds, sliced

Preparation:

- Mix chia seeds with almond milk and let it set in the refrigerator.
- Layer with mixed berries and sliced almonds before serving.

Health Benefits:

- Chia seeds and almonds offer omega-3 fatty acids and antioxidants.

Cooking Time: 5 minutes (plus chilling time)

CONCLUSION

This goal of this Rheumatoid Arthritis Cookbook is to empower individuals with practical and flavorful solutions for managing their health through mindful nutrition. By focusing on anti-inflammatory ingredients, balanced meal plans, and accessible recipes, we've strived to create a resource that not only caters to the unique dietary needs of those with Rheumatoid Arthritis but also inspires a journey towards improved well-being.

Through the exploration of diverse and nutrient-rich recipes, we invite you to embark on a culinary adventure that prioritizes not only the pleasure of the palate but also the nurturing of your body.

The recipes presented here are a testament to the belief that managing Rheumatoid Arthritis can be a holistic and enjoyable endeavor. From the vibrant hues of antioxidant-packed berries to the omega-3-rich embrace of salmon, each ingredient is a deliberate choice aimed at promoting health and flavor in tandem.

As you step into your kitchen armed with this cookbook, remember that the act of preparing and savoring a meal is an act of self-care. It's our hope that these recipes not only provide sustenance for your body but also become a source of joy and empowerment on your journey towards a more vibrant life. May every dish you create be a celebration of your resilience and a nourishing step towards a future filled with well-spiced, wholesome meals and a thriving sense of vitality.

www.ingramcontent.com/pod-product-compliance
Lightning Source LLC
Chambersburg PA
CBHW050834260726

48660CB00006B/2240